Anti-Inflammatory Diet

What the Healthcare Industry Doesn't Want You to Know—Learn How to Cure Autoimmune Diseases and Persistent inflammation for Life Naturally!

Introduction

I want to thank you and congratulate you for downloading the book, *"Anti-Inflammatory Diet: What the Healthcare Industry Doesn't Want You to Know—Learn How to Cure Autoimmune Diseases and Prevent Inflammation for Life Naturally!"*

Have you ever felt like your body just aches and you don't even have any idea why? Have you ever felt bothered because you often suffer from coughs and colds—and it's already making your life like a living hell?

Well, it may be because you are actually suffering from chronic inflammation—a condition that often leads to other ailments or medical conditions that may be the cause of death of most people in the United States alone. So, just imagine what the situation is in other parts of the world!

But, with the help of this book, you'll be able to work on getting yourself out of this rut—so you can go on the path of being a brand new you!

This book contains proven steps and strategies on how to make sure that you start and maintain a healthy diet that will keep you safe from Chronic Inflammation. Read this book now and find out how!

Thanks again for downloading this book, I hope you enjoy it!

TABLE OF CONTENTS

Chapter 1: What Is the Anti-Inflammatory Diet?

The Anti-Inflammatory Diet was originally invented by Dr. Weil, a nutritionist and diet expert. Often said to be almost similar to the Mediterranean Diet and the Zone Diet, but what makes it different is that it involves a lot of fish oil.

The Anti-Inflammatory Diet isn't just about protecting yourself from diseases—it's also about maintaining your ideal weight, too! When you're under this diet, you can expect that you'll easily be able to lose weight in a natural manner.

But what exactly is this about and what could Fish Oil, amongst others, do?

Benefits of Fish Oil

Fish Oil is a good source of Omega-3 Fatty Acids that could strengthen the overall condition of the mind, heart, and immune system in general. This is important because the human body cannot naturally produce Omega-3 Fatty Acids, and a lack of it would therefore bring forth a lot of deficiencies.

More so, one of the main reasons why you need Fish Oil and why the Anti-Inflammatory Diet is around is because it could protect you against Mitochondrial Dysfunction.

Mitochondrial Dysfunction

Mitochondrial Dysfunction results from a combination of erroneous stressors and aging that naturally bring forth a lot of diseases. When a person undergoes this, his cell walls are damaged—which therefore means that he easily becomes susceptible to a lot of negative medical conditions.

Another thing that happens is that free radicals make their way to the body, which then weakens cell membranes, and could bring about heightened levels of Uric Acid that could cause hypertension, slow metabolic rate, and a lot of heart problems.

When these things happen, Chronic Inflammation could take over the body.

Chronic Inflammation

As mentioned earlier, chronic inflammation could be the basis of a lot of dangerous diseases that could ruin the body—mentally, physically, and emotionally. What makes it really scary is the fact that there aren't concrete medical tests that could really check for Chronic Inflammation. Sure, there are cancer tests, heart disease tests, and more, but no one could be able to tell whether you're easily susceptible to these problems or not—and that's why in this case, prevention really proves to be better than cure.

Before you get to know what you should and shouldn't eat, it would be good to first know about what may cause Chronic Inflammation. There are 3 main categories for this, and these are:

1. Physical. This can come from one or more of the following:

Blunt or Penetrating Skin Injuries. It often happens when the injured person picks off scabs from his body.

Burns and Frostbite. These are two extreme effects of the weather, or of accidents that may cause a lot of pain and swelling for the afflicted person.

Debris, dirt, and splinters. Oftentimes, people neglect the way they experience these things and may sometimes be too lazy to take away unnecessary particles from their bodies, and thus, it leads to other diseases and worsening skin conditions.

Ionizing Radiation. There are certain diseases that can be cured by radiation, such as Cancer, but then again, it also has really adverse side effects, such as causing chronic inflammation.

Trauma. When someone gets into a terrible accident, swelling may be induced more and so he may suffer from chronic inflammation.

2. Biological, which is often related to reaction formations in the brain, and could be caused by the following:

Hypersensitivity. Auto-immune Disorders, and other complex immune diseases are often experienced by those who have hypersensitive immune systems.

Pathogenic Infection. Pathogens are microorganisms that may produce certain medical conditions, such as chickenpox, measles, mumps, smallpox, or worse, Ebola.

Stress. When you're stressed, you often experience unusual situations, such as having splotchy skin, feeling depressed, having the worst headaches, and extreme mood swings, which you may think are normal but may mean that certain parts of your body are already in too much pain.

3. Chemical, which are often brought forth by stressors that aren't natural to the body, such as:

Alcohol. Some people's lungs and bodies swell when they drink alcohol.

Irritants. Every person reacts different to irritants that may penetrate their body. Irritants are also called allergens—it could range from pollens, pet fur, legumes, dust mites, spores, or basically anything that makes a person itch, have splotches on the body, and have hard time breathing. You can always ask your doctor for an allergen test so you could determine which allergens you should be aware of.

Toxins. Unfortunately, there are a lot of toxins in the food that one eats and the many drinks around—so you really have to be vigilant and whenever you feel irritated or do not feel normal upon eating or drinking something, feel free to see a doctor already.

Other Factors

Moreover, certain conditions such as having elevated C Proteins, High SED Rate, High Homocystine Levels, Elevated Blood Pressure, and an inhibition of Monocytes could also trigger inflammation rate. It could also be brought upon by:

Age. Age is also a factor. More often than not, people who are in their 30's to 50's and older are more susceptible to this condition, because naturally, younger ones have healthier bodies and tougher immune systems. But then again, everyone's bodies are different so no matter how young you are, you still should not just dismiss this condition as something you won't experience at all. Mitochondrial dysfunction can happen to anyone.

Diet. Mostly, people who are overweight, suffering from Diabetes, and those who consume too much saturated fat are in danger of this.

Excess of Glucose. Glucose is tricky. When they're properly consumed by the body, they can be converted to energy, and the body can use it as its own fuel. But then, an excess of glucose has adverse effects to the body, which may destroy cells and bring forth chronic inflammation, especially when they're just accumulated in the bloodstream.

Low Sex Hormones. Unusual low levels of sex hormones not only kills one's sex life, it may also be the cause of inflammation, and bone breakage. It may also produce unusual symptoms of unease during menopause, as well.

Obesity. As mentioned, being overweight is a problem. When metabolism is affected, it already means that chronic inflammation is happening because the body can no longer secrete and store a lot of hormones and blood circulation is also affected, and thus, cells secrete more fat, which then leads to swelling of the body.

Sleeping Disorders. Pro-inflammatory muscles are elevated when one doesn't have a normal circadian rhythm, and when he almost always has a hard time going to sleep, which is also the result of the elevation of plasma in the body. It also happens to those who has narcolepsy and sleep apnea, too.

Smoking. Inflammation is produced by the thousands of chemicals contained in

Now, when your body gets affected by these things, you can expect that you'd suffer from certain diseases, such as Kawasaki Disease, heart ailments, stroke,

Diabetes, Cancer, Chronic Lower Respiratory Disease, Alzheimer's Disease, Nephritis, and other Autoimmune Diseases.

So, what you have to do then is change your diet and improve your lifestyle—and it all starts with this book.

Chapter 2: Start with the Omegas

As mentioned earlier, your body needs Omega-3 Fatty Acids to function better and to protect you against a wide range of diseases.

When it comes to Omega-3 Fatty Acids, you can't just generalize and say that you'd only be able to get them from salmon, tuna, and other seafood. It's always more than that. There are actually various types of these acids and you can find out more about them below.

Types of Omega-3 Fatty Acids
ALA

ALA, or Alpha Linoleic Acid is a type of fatty acid that's often found in walnuts, seeds, and vegetable oils, most especially soybean, walnuts, hemp, camelina, lingonberry, flax, perilla, kiwi fruit seeds, and chia seeds, amongst others.

ALA is known for the fact that it works in the prevention of prostate cancer and most heart diseases, mostly because its easily synthesized by the body so enzymes could do their work. It is also said that it's best to get your ALA intake from soybeans because their genetic makeup provides so much of it.

DHA

Probably one of the more popular types of fatty acids, DHA stands for Docosahexonic Acid, which is closest to the make-up of the human brain, as well as the retina, testicles, and skin—and that's why it works well with the body. It's also easily synthesized when taken alongside ALA and is known to prevent mental health decline and Alzheimer's Disease, amongst others. Research has it that with the right amount of DHA levels in the brain, mental health decline is lessened by around 45 to 50%.

More so, DHA is also good for pregnant and lactating women—which means that the milk they'd be feeding their babies would be healthy, and would mean that their kids could grow up healthy and strong, too. It also prevents low visual activity, retinal problems, and plasma inconsistencies among children.

DHA also helps in the prevention of cancer, most specifically colon cancer as it decreases the growth of cancer cells and microbes that are found in the said cells.

DHA is usually found in algae supplements, prescription fish oil, orange juice, whole range eggs, fish, and fish oil supplements, amongst others.

EPA

And, finally, you have EPA, which is said to be one of the best types of fatty acid that work with the Anti-Inflammatory Diet.

EPA, which stands for Elcosapentaeonic Acid is a type of fatty acid that naturally lessens inflammation in the body. It is known to be effective in the treatment of common colds and flu, and could also prevent certain medical problems, such as Alzheimer's Disease and schizophrenia, and could also prevent and treat Depression, in some cases. It's also said that when a person is undergoing Chemotherapy, it would be beneficial for him to have some EPA in his system.

You can get EPA from Prescription Fish Oil, Fish Oil Supplements, Whole Range Eggs, Orange Juice, and Fish, amongst others.

Prescription Omega-3s
Meanwhile, if you feel like your Omega-3 intake isn't enough and you don't have the right resources around you, you can ask your doctor for an Omega-3 Prescription.

Once you have a prescription, you can expect your triglyceride levels to be lessened. Triglycerides are a string of enzymes that cause heart diseases and weight gain and that's why it really has to be stopped.

Two of the best types of Prescription Omega-3s are:

Vascepa

Vascepa is often known as Icosapent Ethyl (not Ethyl Alcohol, though) which is usually made from Fish Oil. It easily decreases triglyceride levels and works best when you make some lifestyle changes, such as ending cigarette smoking, and exercising.

Lovaza

There's also something called Lovaza that when used with various types of exercises could actually lower fat levels in the blood, and could help control the body from using other types of drugs. It also increases good cholesterol in the blood, too!

Chapter 3: The Proportions

One thing that you have to understand about the Anti-Inflammatory Diet is that it's all about the proportions. Mainly, it's based on a 2,000 to 3,000 calorie diet, but Dr. Weil said that it will still depend on your age, weight, activity level, and gender, among others.

Main proportions are as follows:

30 Percent – Protein

20 Percent – Fats

40 to 50 Percent – Carbohydrates

Take note that it's important to mix all these ingredients at a given meal so you'd know that you're actually getting the right amount of nutrients that your body needs.

What You Have to Focus On

Aside from Omega-3 Fatty Acids, there are certain types of foods and nutrients that you must include in your daily meals. These are:

Cucumin. Cucumin is often found in an Indian Spice called Turmeric, which is said to be one of the most powerful anti-inflammatory substances that one could find on earth. You can also find cucumin in rosemary and ginger.

Oleic Acid. Oleic Acid is a type of Omega-9 Fatty Acid that could combat chronic ailments by aiding Omega-3 Fatty Acids. When you get a combination of these acids, your body begins to react in such a way that it learns how to adapt to certain situations, making it not susceptible to diseases. You can mostly get Oleic Acid from Olive Oil—which can be used for healthy cooking, Macadamias, and Almonds.

Antioxidants. Antioxidants fight free radicals—giving you a healthy, natural glow. And because they get to fight free radicals, you can expect that your body will be able to fight chronic diseases, too. Most fruits and vegetables are rich in antioxidants, but you could get it mostly from Kale, Spinach, Vitamin C, Bell Peppers, Beta-Carotene, Winter Squash, and Oranges.

Quercetin. This one is a natural anti-histamine—so it's perfect for those who suffer from Asthma and allergic reactions. It is also known as the best kind of flavonoid. The best sources include apples, broccoli, onions, and red grapes.

Polyphenols. Polyphencls naturally dampen the existence of phytochemicals that cause inflammation. They also prevent oxidation disruption and can be found mostly in raspberries, strawberries, blackberries, blueberries, and other colorful fruits.

To give you a better idea about how to go forth with this diet, read on and understand that there are various types of foods that you could eat—and of course, some of them you could eat in unlimited amounts while you can eat the rest on a controlled manner.

Unlimited Amounts

First, you have foods that you can eat in unlimited amounts, and this includes herbs, spices, and Asian Mushrooms. Take note that:

1. You should never eat mushrooms raw, because they may be poisonous.

2. Only eat commercial mushrooms such as Crimini or Portobello in minimal amounts. It's always best to eat mushrooms such as Shitake, Enokidake, Oyster, and Wild, as well.

3. Asian Mushrooms are always the best because they contain lots of anti-inflammatory compounds that improves digestion and strengthens the immune system as a whole.

4. As for herbs and spices, it's best to add turmeric, curry powder, thyme, garlic, ginger, chili powder, cinnamon, and rosemary into your dishes. Herbs and Spices are important not only because they protect your body from most diseases, but also because they could improve your metabolic rate—so you could reach your ideal weight in time!

5 to 7 times a Day

Then, you have healthy fats which you can eat for around 5 to 7 times in a day. For these, you have to remember that:

1. One whole serving of healthy fats may mean a combination of a teaspoon of oil, 2 walnuts, a tablespoon of flaxseed, and an ounce of avocado.

2. You can also consider foods rich in Omega-3 Fatty Acids as an example of healthy fat. Refer to Chapter 2 for more information about this.

4 to 5 times a Day

Next, there are foods you have to eat for at least 4 to 5 times in a day. In this case, you have vegetables and so you have to remember that:

1. A good example of a serving of vegetables is a combination of raw or juiced vegetables, ½ cup cooked vegetables, and at least 2 cups of salad greens.

2. Best choices include washed raw salad greens, sea vegetables, squashes, peas, onions, beets, carrots, cauliflower, bok choy, kale, Brussels sprouts, cabbage, broccoli, Swiss Chard, collard greens, and spinach.

3. Organic vegetables are better than other types.

4. Vegetables are big part of the anti-inflammatory diet because they naturally have anti-inflammatory and anti-oxidant properties, mainly because they contain flavonoids and carotenoids.

5. You can eat vegetables whether they're raw or cooked.

3 to 5 times a Day

1. Whole and Cracked Grains can then be eaten 3 to 5 times a day. For this category, you have to take note that:

2. ½ cup cooked grains is an example of one serving of this food group.

3. Best choices include steel-cut oats, basmati rice, bulgur, muesli, groats, buckwheat, wild rice, and brown rice.

4. Products made from flour and whole wheat bread are not whole grains. Take note that whole grains are those that are in large pieces or that are intact.

5. Whole grains are perfect because they metabolize in such a way that blood sugar doesn't spike and so inflammation is prevented from happening.

3 to 4 times a Day

As for fruits, you can have them at least 3 to 4 times each day. Just remember that:

1. A prime example of 1 serving of fruits would be a combination of ½ cup dried fruit, ½ cup chopped fruit, and a medium piece of fruit, as well.

2. Best choices include pears, apples, cherries, blackberries, pomegranates, plums, red grapes, pink grapefruit, oranges, nectarines, peaches, strawberries, blueberries, and raspberries.

3. Just like vegetables, fruits also have anti-oxidant and anti-inflammatory properties mainly because of carotenoids and flavonoids. Make sure to go for organic and choose as much colors as you want.

2 to 4 times a Day

If you're fond of drinking, why not drink tea, instead? You can have it for at least 2 to 4 times in a day alone. Just take note that:

1. Inflammation is reduced because tea contains catechins that naturally fight inflammation and strengthen the immune system, as well.

2. Oolong, green, and white tea are the best choices.

1 to 2 times a Day

Meanwhile, you can have 1 to 2 servings of legumes and beans each day—unless you have rheumatoid arthritis. You could also take red wine in the same amount. Just remember that:

1. ½ cup cooked legumes or beans is an example of one serving of this food group.

2. Beans and legumes contain lots of soluble fiber, potassium, magnesium, and folic acid which can easily break down glucose and protect the body from most diseases.

3. Best choices include lentils, black-eyed peas, chickpeas, adzuki, and Anasazi beans.

4. When consumed in moderation, you can also benefit from red wine because of its anti-oxidant properties.

2 to 6 times a Week

Now, you should also make sure to eat fish and seafood 2 to 6 times in a week. For this, you have to take note that:

1. 4 oz of seafood or fish is a prime example of 1 serving of this food group.

2. Best choices include sablefish, salmon, black cod, sardines, and herring.

3. However, if you do not like fish, keep in mind that fish-oil supplements will do, as long as you take at least 2 to 3 grams of them each day.

4. The right fish and seafood have anti-inflammatory properties because they're rich in Omega-3 Fatty Acids.

2 to 3 times a Week

As for pasta, you can have it at least 2 to 3 times each week. Take note that:

1. ½ cup cooked pasta is an example of 1 serving of this food group.

2. Best choices include Japanese Soba, Udon, Buckwheat Noodles, part whole wheat noodles, bean thread noodles, organic pasta.

3. When cooked al-dente, pasta gets a low glycemic index and does a lot of good for your blood glucose levels.

1 to 2 times a Week

As mentioned earlier, you also need some protein in your system—and you should include other types of proteins in your diet and have them at least once or twice a week. Remember that:

1. An example of 1 serving of this food group is a combination of 3 oz skinless meat or cooked poultry, 1 egg, one 8 oz serving of dairy, as well as an ounce of cheese.

2. Best choices include grass-fed lean meats, skinless poultry, Omega-3 enriched eggs, yogurt, and natural cheese.

Eat Sparingly

And of course, there are certain types of food that you should just eat sparingly, and these are called healthy sweets. Remember that:

1. Best choices include fruit sorbet, dark chocolate, and unsweetened dried fruit.

2. Chocolates have anti-oxidant properties because they contain polyphenols. This way, you'd look and feel radiant.

Vitamins and Supplements

There are also some vitamins and supplements that you can take to aid you in this diet. These include:

Vitamin A. This helps in the prevention of diseases that affect the kidneys and the liver, as well as lung diseases, acne, and inflammatory bowel syndrome, as well. It's mostly found in green leafy vegetables and carrots. An increase of Vitamin A in your system could also protect you from those free radicals, too.

Vitamin B6. Vitamin 6 is amazing because it's water soluble—so it means that it's easily absorbed by the body. It's usually found in fish, vegetables, and lean meat such as turkey. Without Vitamin B6, you could be afflicted with rheumatoid arthritis and heart diseases.

Vitamin C. Vitamin C has natural healing components, so of course, that reduces the risk of inflammation. Aside from that, it also improves collagen buildup. When this happens, you can expect that your blood vessels, ligaments, cartilage, and arteries will be stronger, and apart from that, Vitamin C could also lessen the amount of C-Reactive Proteins in your body, too.

Vitamin D. Vitamin D lessens inflammation and strengthens the bones. It's usually found in most fortified foods, egg yolks, beef, liver, eggs, and fish. It protects you against Rickets, Inflammatory Bowel Disease, Lupus, and Arthritis, as well as other age-related diseases, and reduced the risk of colon cancer by at least 40%.

Vitamin E. Vitamin E could help you look good as it is a natural antioxidant. And of course, when you look good, you could expect that you'd feel good, too. Aside from that, it also protects the body against heart diseases and could also combat most allergies. You can get it mostly from green leafy vegetables, seeds, and nuts.

Vitamin K. Vitamin K is essential in the proper clotting of the blood and is mostly found in green leafy vegetables, broccoli, and asparagus. It's also said to improve inflammatory protection in general.

What to Avoid

Meanwhile, you also have to make sure that you get to avoid foods such as beef, yeast, milk, and most dairy by-products. This is because these foods often just burn the body from the inside. In other words, they cause inflammation. You can also take a look at the list below to see what you shouldn't add in your grocery list:

2% or Whole Milk. Too much of this is bad because it is high in saturated fat, which of course, causes inflammation.

Alcohol. Alcohol is one big irritant, especially if you're naturally allergic to it or if you've already had too much, because bacteria passes through the intestinal linings easily. Also, alcohol instantly becomes sugar once it has gone through the process of metabolism.

Cheeseburgers. They're really tasty, but then they can also do a lot of wrong for your body. Burgers are full of saturated fat that break down the gut and make it hard for you to keep your body safe from various diseases.

Gluten. When there's too much gluten in your body, swelling will be prevalent.

MSG. The body isn't used to MSG, and that's why it's also said that eating junk foods, such as chips and other salty food products can do a lot of damage to the body.

Omega-6 Fatty Acids. Too much of these, especially those coming from legumes, may make chronic inflammation prevalent.

Too much sugar. Too much sugar means there'd be excessive amounts of glucose in your body, too, and as mentioned earlier, this isn't very ideal.

White Bread. White bread is a prime source of carbohydrates that are easily broken down into sugar which again, turns into glucose. Too much of it cannot be turned into fuel so the body will definitely suffer.

Chapter 4: Customize the Diet

What was given in the earlier chapter is of course, a general guideline about the Anti-Inflammatory Diet. Because there are various types of health problems that people face, you could also expect that the diet would have different restrictions for these situations. As for that, you can keep in mind the following:

Anti-Diabetic Diet

The Anti-Inflammatory Diet is close to Mediterranean and Vegetarian Diets which are recommended for people who have diabetes, or for those who want to prevent diabetes from happening.

If you want to tweak it even more, you could add make use of superfoods that are great against Diabetes and most health problems. These include yogurt, fat-free milk, nuts, whole grains, fish, tomatoes, berries, sweet potatoes, citrus fruits, and dark green leafy vegetables. Never go for packaged meals—make sure to prepare your meals by yourself.

Gluten-Free Diet

The Anti-Inflammatory Diet is also very friendly to those under or who want to try the Gluten-Free Diet. You can only just focus on quinoa or rice and avoid unhealthy grains, such as rye, barley, and wheat.

Vegan and Vegetarian

Again, this is primarily based on vegetables so one could just cut back on their intake of meats and carbohydrates. If one's Pesco-Vegetarian, he could also eat fish and seafood so he'd have some Omega-3 intake. Otherwise, he could just ask the doctor for Omega-3 supplement prescriptions.

Kosher Diet

If you're Jewish, you could also pattern the anti-inflammatory diet to your beliefs. Mostly, you can eat potatoes or sweet potatoes, vegetables, fruits, and stay away from meat. So again, there wouldn't be a big problem for you.

Low-Salt

You also wouldn't have a problem with this because fruits and vegetables are naturally low in salt in the first place.

Chapter 5: What Else Should You Expect?

And finally, here are the other things that you could expect when it comes to this diet.

Is it easy to follow?

Well, what you have to keep in mind is that nothing's really that easy to follow. But, if you put your heart and mind and commit yourself to one thing then it would be easy for you.

As for the Anti-Inflammatory Diet, it's actually not that difficult to follow because meal plans aren't very restrictive, in a sense that there aren't really "meal plans" that you have to follow. As mentioned earlier, you can customize it according to your lifestyle, just as long as you follow guidelines about what you can and cannot eat. Again, that would be a lot of fruits, vegetables, and fish oil—and the rest can follow.

You can buy fruits and vegetables in your local groceries or markets, so that wouldn't be a problem. Fish Oil is also becoming popular so pretty sure that you can get a hold of it without any problem, too.

Is it affordable?

Fruits and Vegetables do not cost too much. Most food products that contain Fish Oil are quite affordable, as well. Supplements would of course cost a bit higher than them, but nothing that would burn a big hole in your pocket.

You can also buy cookbooks from the internet, or from Dr. Weil's website, if you really want to see Anti-Inflammatory Recipes. Just prepare around $1.99 to $29.99 and you're set.

Will it taste good?

The good thing about most healthy diets these days is the fact that food actually tastes good; it's never bland and wouldn't make you feel like you just don't want to eat at all. In fact, out of those vegetables you could create your own versions of pasta. Or, you can try making various salads or even snacks, such as Kale chips. And, because you're allowed to use herbs and seasonings, you can really take it up a notch and let those dishes satisfy your tastebuds!

Will you be satiated enough?

Another great thing about the Anti-Inflammatory Diet is that since it's based on the 2000 to 3000 calorie diet, it would definitely leave you satiated and because you'd have all these fruits and vegetables, you could also expect that your body will be filled with fiber. When this happens, hunger will be staved off—so you wouldn't feel the need to eat over and over and over again.

Is it convenient?

Yes, because the dishes would be really good. Again, you can check various cookbooks and Dr. Weil's official one for this, but generally, it is quite convenient. What only makes it inconvenient is the time you'll be spending for preparing the meals. But, don't worry because you can always eat outside –just as long as you remember the types of food that you have to avoid.

In this case, you have to make sure that you check out the menus of the restaurants you'll be eating at, or check their websites, if possible. This way, you'd know what you should expect right away. Take note that you could actually drink alcohol, but it would be best to keep it in moderation. Don't go over 1 to 2 glasses each night!

Dr. Weil says that you could always go for Japanese Food—so if you're fond of that, then you'd have no problems with this diet.

And, should you exercise?

While Dr. Weil didn't really put exercise as part of the Anti-Inflammatory Diet, you should still keep in mind that exercising regularly is a good part of any diet and of any lifestyle. When you exercise regularly, you'd feel so much better about yourself—and so the diet that you're in could work for you even better!

Keep these things in mind and you'll surely be on the right track!

Conclusion

It is becoming increasingly clear that chronic inflammation is the root cause of many serious illnesses - including heart disease, many cancers, and alzheimer's disease. We all know inflammation on the surface of the body as local redness, heat, swelling and pain. It is the cornerstone of the body's healing response, bringing more nourishment and more immune activity to a site of injury or infection. But when inflammation persists or serves no purpose, it damages the body and causes illness. Stress, lack of exercise, genetic predisposition, and exposure to toxins (like secondhand tobacco smoke) can all contribute to such chronic inflammation, but dietary choices play a big role as well. Learning how specific foods influence the inflammatory process is the best strategy for containing it and reducing long-term disease risks.

The Anti-Inflammatory Diet is not a diet in the popular sense - it is not intended as a weight-loss program (although people can and do lose weight on it), nor is it an eating plan to stay on for a limited period of time. Rather, it is way of selecting and preparing foods based on scientific knowledge of how they can help your body maintain optimum health. Along with influencing inflammation, this diet will provide steady energy and ample vitamins, minerals, essential fatty acids dietary fiber, and protective phytonutrients.

Thank you and good luck!

Check out my other Best Selling Books Below!!

Preview From Best Selling Author Jessica Virna "Hormone Reset Diet"

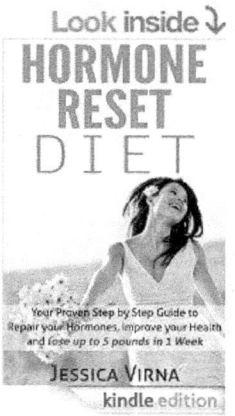

Chapter 1: Hormonal Imbalance: The Root Cause of Weight Loss Problems

Have you ever wondered why none of the dietary programs you have tried really worked well for you? Do you still gain weight despite all your hard work in keeping yourself fit? Do you easily feel stressed out with simple things? If you answered "yes" to all these questions, then you have failed to address the real root cause of the problem—hormonal imbalance.

Here are some questions that you need to ask yourself first to help determine if you have imbalanced hormones or not:

- Do you usually feel a strong urge to eat sweets or carbs at 3pm?
- Do you find it difficult to get yourself out of bed in the morning?
- Do you easily get irritated even by simple things?
- Do have mood swings?
- Do you experience pre-menstrual syndrome every month?
- Do you have trouble getting a good night's sleep?
- Is your skin dull and dry?
- Do you have a belly fat that you can't seem to get rid of no matter what you do?
- Do you always feel bloated after every meal?

If your answer is "yes" to all of these questions, then your hormone levels are not balanced. Fortunately, this book was written specifically for you.

Women are more susceptible to problems pertaining to hormones. No matter how little we eat or how healthy our diet is, if it doesn't balance out hormonal misfires then the efforts will be wasted for nothing. There are different signs of hormonal imbalances and often women fail to recognize that.

- Pre-menstrual syndrome
- Irritability and mood swings over little things
- Extra weight hanging around the waist/belly area
- Excessive cravings for sugar
- Easily stressed out
- Difficulty sleeping
- Overwhelming feeling

Women need to know that hormones control nearly all aspects of losing weight. They affect your appetite, food cravings, fat storage, food patterns and even gut bacteria. This means that when there's hormonal imbalance, nothing will work out well for you unless you address this problem first. Eliminating junk foods and exercising regularly have always been the experts' advice on losing weight, but with hormones getting all fired up, losing weight will be difficult.

Click Here to Check out the Rest of "The Hormone Reset Diet" on Amazon

Or go to: **http://amzn.to/1HhshKh**

Preview Of "Mediterranean Diet"

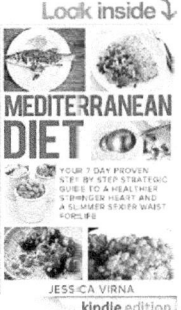

Chapter 1 Benefits of the Mediterranean Diet

There is a renewed attention and enthusiasm about the Mediterranean diet in recent years. A lot of researches found out that the diet is rich in nuts, fresh vegetables and fruits, olive oil and fish, providing protection against serious illnesses. Aside from that, it also helps in maintaining a healthy weight.

More specific health benefits include:

Protection from Type 2 Diabetes

Traditional Mediterranean diet is rich in fiber. The fiber slows down the rate of digestion of carbohydrates. This way, the blood sugar levels do not quickly shoot up and just as rapidly drop. Type 2 diabetes develops from rapid sugar-insulin spikes that occur frequently.

Protects against stroke and heart diseases

Modern, average meals are high in processed food and red meat. All these contribute to increasing one's risk in developing stroke and cardiovascular diseases. All these food are highly discouraged in the Mediterranean diet. Also, red wine is more preferred than drinking hard liquor. Research studies showed that red wine contains beneficial compounds that provide protective effects on the heart and the cardiovascular system.

Reduced risk of developing Parkinson's disease

The diet provides a substantial amount of antioxidants obtained from the abundance of fresh fruits and vegetables. These antioxidants provide a protective effect on the cells against damage from oxidative stress. Parkinson's disease develops from the degeneration or destruction of the nerve cells. By taking more antioxidants, the cells will have better protection against destruction. This also helps reduce the risk of Parkinson's by as much as 50%.

Reduced risk of developing Alzheimer's disease

Research found that following a Mediterranean diet improves the body's lipid profile. It improves the levels of cholesterol in the blood and promotes better ration between LDL and HDL. Also, blood sugar levels are better regulated. All these improvements are believed by experts to help in reducing a person's risk for developing Alzheimer's disease.

Reduced risk for cancers

Healthier eating practices help in preventing several types of cancer. Increased fiber intake helps reduce colon cancers. Antioxidants from fresh fruits and vegetables help in strengthening the cells against damage and cancer formation.

Vitamins and minerals help the body's organs to repair itself and recover faster and better, to prevent any cancer cells from developing within the damaged structures.

Improved musculoskeletal health

The diet is rich in natural vitamins, minerals and other essential nutrients that help keep the joints, muscle and the rest of the musculoskeletal system working well and free of pain. A study found that the nutrients supplied by the Mediterranean diet helps in reducing the elderly's risk for muscle weakness and frailty symptoms related to advancement of age.

Longer life

Because of the reduced risk for diseases such as cancer and heart attack, a person has a 20% reduction in death risk. That is, those who follow the Mediterranean diet enjoy longer, healthier lives.

Weight loss

All these healthy eating practices help lose excess weight and maintain it within the healthy range. Numerous researches on obesity found that frequent sugar and insulin spikes promote fat accumulation in the body and slow down metabolism and fat burning. Unhealthy trans fats and saturated fats from the average diet are not utilized by the body and are stored as added fats. Also, the chemicals from food processing such as the preservatives, flavor enhancers and stabilizers all contribute to an imbalance in the body that promotes obesity. Take all these out and the body is able to return to its normal and efficient metabolism and fat control. The net result is losing excess weight.

Click Here to Check out The Rest of "The Mediterranean Diet" on Amazon

Or go to: **http://amzn.to/1e1YtVA**

Preview From Best Selling Author Jessica Virna "The Truth About Carbs"

Look inside ↓

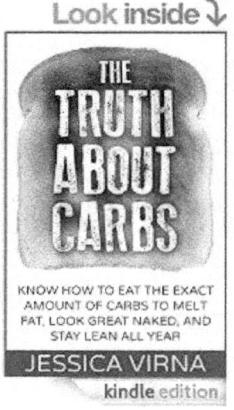

Introduction

I want to thank you and congratulate you for downloading the book, *"The Truth About Carbs: Know How To Eat The Exact Amount Of Carbs To Melt Fat, Look Great Naked, And Stay Lean All Year."*

So many have tried countless dieting regimes — detox, vegan, Paleo, South Beach, etc. — but many had not yet met success in terms of weight loss and achieving a leaner, slimmer figure. What could be the problem? While the ultimate goal is to lose weight, some people have trouble losing *fat*. This book is aimed toward those dieters and anyone who wants to learn how to melt fat and stay lean, by focusing on the ever-elusive, ever-controversial *carbohydrates*.

This book will teach you the *truth* about carbs and how you can deal with this molecule. You don't have to *completely eliminate* carbs and say goodbye to your favorite food groups (never say goodbye to pastries or pasta!). You will learn how to eat carbs the proper way — for the benefit of your health and the success of your fat-loss endeavor.

Click here to check out the Rest of "The Truth About Carbs" on Amazon

Or go to: http://amzn.to/1RFykvc

Preview From Best Selling Author Jessica Virna "Essential Oils Therapy"

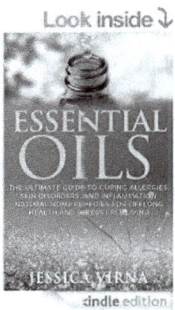

Benefits of Aromatherapy

There are various benefits of aromatherapy and possess different properties. Even if essential oils are good for first aid and relief, they are not enough to take the place of professional medication from licensed healthcare practitioners. Likewise, it is always good measure to have a person checked after providing first aid.

Essential oils can be unassuming but can have many versatile uses in a household. It pays to familiarize yourself with properties of essential oils so that you can act fast and know what needs to be done in case of emergencies.

Benefits

1. Improves skin
2. Helps digestion
3. Promotes sleep and relaxation
4. Natural first aid
5. Aromatherapy

Properties

1. Analgesic-some essential oils can relieve pain such as lavender, black pepper and bergamot.

2. Anesthetic-for emergencies, peppermint, clove, bay and eucalyptus can be used as an anaesthetic.

3. Antimicrobial-anise, bay, cajuput and benzoin along with black pepper have the ability to destroy or suppress microorganism and bacterial growth.

4. Antioxidant-essential oils can help remove damaging oxidizing agents in the body like ginger and benzoin.

5. Antiseptic-there are essential oils that can prevent decay like basil, bay, cedarwood, cinnamon, pine, sage, thyme and ylang ylang.

6. Antispasmodic-clove, cypress, garlic, thyme and basil essential oils can relive the nerves and reduce or prevent excessive muscular spasms and contractions.

7. Carminative-carminative properties mean that an essential oil has the ability to stimulate intestinal peristalsis, and relieve the expulsion of gas from the gastrointestinal tract. Such is the use of cinnamon, coriander, garlic, lemon, black pepper, basil and anise because they tend to introduce *heat* in the body.

8. Disinfectant-there are natural disinfectants in the organic world and the citrus essential oils are always dual purpose, like lemon and orange because of their acidic properties.

9. Stimulant-stimulants increase functional activity and energy in the body, which essential oils like bergamot, juniper, peppermint, jasmine and thyme can do.

10. Tonic- tonics tend to energize and strengthen the body like thyme, yarrow, black pepper, eucalyptus and cajuput.

Essential oils are more than just a good scent and home décor. There are many health benefits that can be derived from these natural wonders. Use your imagination and live a healthier lifestyle, you definitely deserve it.

Click Here to check out the Rest of "Essential Oils Therapy" on Amazon

Or Go to: http://amzn.to/1cUvAdI

Preview From Best Selling Author Jessica Virna "Weight Watchers"

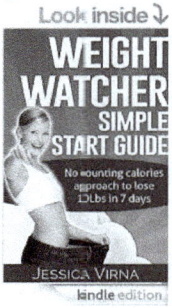

Chapter 1. Weight Watchers and PointsPlus Value

The Weight Watchers® diet program is centered on food that is low in fat but high in fiber. Eat a lot of food within this selection in order to lose 1 to 2 pounds a day. There are times when you may crave for high fat muffins; the Weight Watcher recipes included in this cookbook has low fat and delicious muffins for you to prepare.

This diet program focuses on fruits, vegetables and protein that will enable you to increase your energy. Spend the energy at the gym to gain muscles instead of sitting on a couch the whole day.

Losing 10 lbs. in a week will not be difficult at all! The Weight Watchers® program now boasts of its new and improved PointsPlus values that will guide you to balance your food intake to lose weight. Based on a 1,000 calorie/day diet, you will learn how to eat a filling and balanced meal. Within the PointsPlus directives, you are allowed to consume 26 to 71 points in a day.

Keep in mind that you are not required to eat within the maximum limits that the point guide suggests. This is to give you a non-restrictive diet plan that will not leave you weak while in the process of losing weight.

Physical activity is needed to burn the extra calories that you have gained should you reach the maximum limits of the Weight Watchers® provisionary PointsPlus. In order for you to effectively lose weight, why not try to splurge more on fruits and vegetable? For you see, they have a PointsPlus value of 0. This way, you will feel full without having to think about the calories.

Among the Weight Watchers® dieters, this technique is called the filling technique. They eat designated food that does not add weight and calories. To bring the PointsPlus calorie tracker to a mathematical explanation, you simply would have to allocate points depending on your weight, height, activity level and age.

Aside from the PointsPlus® formula which can be calculated through a link in the website, there is also the ActivityPoints formula wherein you can check as to how many points you can include in your meal plan; based on the level of your physical activities. The more active you are, the higher your PointsPlus allocation is.

Keeping the weight off will not be a problem at all through the help of the Weight Watchers PointsPlus technique. This cookbook will show you the healthy way that the author chose to follow in order to lose 140 lbs.

<u>Click Here to check out the Rest of "Weight Watchers Guide"</u>

Or go to: **http://amzn.to/1G75fnI**

Preview From Best Selling Author Jessica Virna "Buddhism"

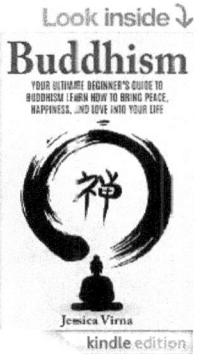

The First Noble Truth: Suffering

The enlightened Buddha realized that life is full of suffering. Whether one looks at his own life or at the world around him, this state is inescapable. The Buddha saw the world of suffering the moment he left the palace. In fact, the pre-conditions to fulfill the prophecy all pointed to different forms of suffering. Through the old man, he saw that everyone would eventually suffer of old age. One's former complexion may fade and wrinkles would surface. His strength would diminish; his capabilities would lessen.

The image of the sick man also portrayed the reality of people being prone to illnesses and diseases. Despite the joys of being healthy, this state wouldn't always be present. One's eyes may begin having difficulty seeing and other body parts may experience pain that wasn't formerly present. Moreover, death could strike anyone at any minute. In seeing the image of the funeral, Siddhartha saw that everyone would experience death.

For someone who was never exposed to pain, all these realities can be very overwhelming. From the moment a child is born until his death, pain would be present. However, these didn't cause Siddhartha to lock himself up in the palace. In fact, the words of the hermit even inspired him to discover more about suffering in the hopes of learning how to achieve happiness.

The first noble truth embraces the inevitability of suffering. Despite the joys and pleasures of life, pain would always appear. However, despite the negativity that this may indicate, the Buddha explains that these are normal. These should not be feared or hated. Rather, people must accept suffering and prepare for it.

Knowing Suffering

Suffering can come in two main forms. First, there is physical pain. This can be seen through harm inflicted on the body. Wounds, fractured legs, or even sickness are indicators of physical harm. Such suffering can be of varying degrees. They can last for as little as a few seconds to even an entire lifetime. However, while most people view suffering to be applicable only to the physical body, the Buddha clarified that this can also emerge in the spirit.

People experience various emotions. These include hate, anger, and greed. People can even feel depressed or lonely. Many of these are unhealthy and unwanted feelings that can affect one's health and disposition. The death of loved ones and other unfortunate events can also trigger such hardships and emotions. Failures and losses can also result to this painful sensation. While these emotions seem to be hidden and minor, they can cause worse effects than physical pain. In fact, they can even elevate the suffering caused by the physical body.

Although people want to experience as little pain as possible, it is clear that this would exist in everyday situations. Even the most minor nuances can trigger suffering. However, the Buddha teaches his followers that these are all natural. Instead of fearing or running away from such emotions, one should slowly and carefully learn to accept these. In fact, knowing suffering would be the key to eventually know happiness.

Of Suffering and Happiness

Although suffering is dominant in life, the Buddha also claims that joy and happiness can also be found simultaneously. Amidst the pain, there can be happiness in friendship, family, health, and other positive factors. These would depend on the perception of an individual. While there are times for suffering, there would also be times of happiness. Buddhists would claim that while both are part of life, these aren't necessarily present permanently. There is some form of balance which can be handled by individuals.

Knowing that suffering and happiness can coexist, the Buddhists proceed to explain that many people make the mistake of trying to escape suffering. They try to distract themselves by indulging in temporary pleasure. Drinking, gambling, and other habits are methods to forget about these unwanted feelings. In their attempt to block out sadness, loss, and grief, they try to delude themselves with pleasure. However, in reality, these wouldn't be effective and would just end up bringing more severe forms of pain and sadness. This would produce worse effects once the temporary happiness perishes. For example, if a person with a cold tries to cheer himself up by eating ice cream, this may just temporarily satisfy his taste buds. After a while, this would contribute to the worsening condition of his colds.

Applying the First Noble Truth

It is important to accept the first truth if one desires to be a step closer to knowing how to gain happiness and enlightenment. Although this teaching may be ancient, this is very applicable to this day and age.

1) It's okay to be worried, but don't let it control your life.

People may get the misconception that the first truth encourages them to stop worrying about bills, insurance, and other things. However, this is incorrect. Fear caused by possible suffering is normal. After all, it's an undesirable state to be in. One shouldn't become boastful and feel invincible to suffering. However, at the same time, one shouldn't let the emotions inflicted by suffering take control of his life. Instead of letting it dictate one's disposition, it should help strengthen one's morale and character. Yes, suffering can sometimes feel too unbearable. However, suffering will always be merely a state that can be overcome. Hence, there is a need to control one's emotions. In effect, he can live life more fully and strive to find happiness.

2) Prepare for suffering. It will always be there.

One shouldn't just offer himself to suffering. Of course, he should find ways to prepare for it or even prevent it from worsening. An individual can choose to plan ahead, ask help from friends, or other methods to cater to his needs. He doesn't have to face suffering unarmed.

3) Be optimistic.

Many people who experience suffering feel as if it indicates the end of the world. They may lose the will to work or even live. These thoughts won't be beneficial in one's pursuit of happiness. Suffering is perfectly normal. Though suffering may hinder a person to fulfill his goals or plans, this doesn't mean that suffering should take control of the rest of his life. One should still think positive amidst the pain he endures. This perhaps is the most effective way to combat such feelings.

4) Be realistic.

Suffering is very real and shouldn't be taken for granted. Hence, one should understand how it can affect his life. Knowing the implications of a certain form of suffering can be helpful as one responds to it. Understanding a certain health illness or consequences of not paying bills can all help the person experiencing problems.

For the Buddha, there is a need to focus on the realities of life. To achieve happiness, one must embrace whatever is happening in life. Distractions would be of temporary benefit but would be inevitably futile. Hence, as both happiness and suffering are both temporary, people must learn to live with these. This is the first step to achieving inner peace and enlightenment. Of course, it doesn't end there. The Buddha then proceeds to discuss the succeeding truths.

Click **Here** to check out the Rest of "BUDDHISM: Your Ultimate Beginner's Guide to Bring Peace, Happiness, and Enlightenment Into Your Daily Life" on Amazon

Or Go To: http://amzn.to/1QK7j8r

Preview Of 'Insert Book Title Here'

This section is designed to provide the reader a preview of one of your other books. Simply copy and paste a chapter of another book that you have available on Kindle and link to it below.

Click here to check out the rest of (insert book name here) on Amazon.

Or go to: **http://www.mybitlylink.com** (insert shortened bit.ly link)